The Red Light Therapy Handbook
Techniques, Benefits, and Applications

James Peterson

Copyright@2024 James Peterson all right Reserved, No part of this publication may be reproduced in any form or means without prior written permission from the copyright holder

Chapter One

Definition and Fundamental principle of red light Therapy

Chapter Two

The Science Behind Red Light Therapy

Chapter Three

Technique on How to Begin Red Light Therapy Treatment

Chapter Four

Application Techniques Comparing Indirect and Direct Applications

Chapter Five

Red Light Therapy in Combination with Other Therapies Treatment

Chapter Six

Benefits of red light therapy Skin Care and Beauty

Chapter Seven

Red Light Therapy at Home

Chapter Eight

Commonly Asked Questions Generally Questions

Chapter One

Definition and Fundamental principle of red light Therapy

Red light therapy (RLT) is a therapeutic approach that uses particular wavelengths of red and near-infrared light to enhance cellular function and healing. It is also referred to as low-level laser therapy (LLLT), photobiomodulation (PBM), or cold laser therapy. The therapy entails exposing the skin to low levels of these wavelengths of light, which can penetrate the skin and be absorbed by the cells.

Historical Background and Evolution

- **Ancient Origins:** The Greeks, Egyptians, and Romans employed sunlight's curative qualities, a procedure known as heliotherapy, to treat their ailments.
- **Modern Discovery:** In the middle of the 20th century, Hungarian physician Endre Mester conducted research with low-level lasers and found that certain wavelengths of light may be therapeutic. In 1967, Mester also found that low-level lasers could promote hair growth and wound healing.
- **Device Development:** In the last few decades, technological

developments have prompted the creation of a wide range of red light therapy devices, from at-home gadgets to specialized hospital equipment.

Goals and Purpose of the Book

This book covers the science behind red light therapy, practical application techniques, the wide range of benefits, and various real-world applications. It is intended for a wide audience, including healthcare professionals, therapists, athletes, and individuals seeking alternative methods for health and wellness. The goal of this book is to provide a comprehensive guide to understanding and using red light therapy.

- **Educational Resource:** To inform readers about red light therapy's workings, advantages, and safe applications.
- **Practical Guide:** To offer detailed guidelines and procedures for applying red light treatment in different contexts.
- **Research and Case Studies:** To provide fact-based data and actual case studies demonstrating the efficacy of red light treatment.
- **Future Insights:** To investigate new directions in the

field, current studies, and the prospects for red light treatment in the fields of health and wellbeing.

By the time they finish reading this book, readers will have a solid understanding of red light therapy's operation, practical use, and range of health and wellbeing benefits.

Chapter Two

The Science Behind Red Light Therapy

How Cellular Red Light Therapy Operates

Red and near-infrared light are applied topically to the body as part of red light treatment (RLT). The light permeates the skin and is absorbed by cells, stimulating a variety of biological processes:

• **Photon Absorption:** A number of biological processes are triggered when red or near-infrared light photons are absorbed by chromophores within cells, especially by cytochrome c oxidase in the mitochondria.

- **ATP creation:** Light absorption increases the efficiency of the mitochondrial respiratory chain, which in turn increases the creation of adenosine triphosphate (ATP), the cell's energy currency. This increase in ATP production gives cells more energy to carry out their activities efficiently.
- **Reactive Oxygen Species (ROS):** Moderate exposure to red light can induce mild oxidative stress, which in turn produces ROS. This type of regulated stress promotes cellular defense systems and repair without causing harm to the cells.

The Function of ATP Production and Mitochondria

• **Mitochondrial Function**: Often referred to as the "powerhouses of the cell," mitochondria are vital for energy production and cellular metabolism. Red light therapy helps cells produce more ATP by enhancing mitochondrial function, which is necessary for cell growth, repair, and maintenance.

• **Cellular Respiration:** Higher levels of mitochondrial activity contribute to more effective cellular respiration, which is essential for the general well-being and the operation of tissues and organs. This is especially true for cells found in tissues with high energy requirements, like muscles, the brain, and the skin.

Important Wavelengths and Their Function

The two main wavelength ranges used in red light treatment are the red (600–700 nm) and near-infrared (700–1100 nm). Each wavelength range has advantages and consequences of its own.

- **Red Light (600–700nm):**
- **Skin Health:** This product works wonders for skin issues like acne, scars, and wrinkles by penetrating the skin to improve collagen synthesis, reduce inflammation, and enhance wound healing.

- **Surface-Level Benefits:** Good for ailments and treatments at the surface, with comparatively quick noticeable outcomes.
- **Near-Infrared Light (700–1100 nm):**
- **Deep Tissue Penetration:** This type of treatment is useful for treating musculoskeletal difficulties, lowering pain, and improving muscle recovery since it penetrates deeper into the body, reaching muscles, joints, and even bones.
- **Pain reduction and Inflammation Reduction:** It helps with ailments including tendinitis, arthritis, and muscle strains by promoting anti-

inflammatory effects and pain reduction in deeper tissues.

Biological effect

- **Enhanced Blood Flow:** Red light therapy induces vasodilation, which improves tissue oxygenation and blood flow. This aids in the delivery of vital nutrients and the elimination of waste materials from cells.

- **Anti-Inflammatory Actions:** Red light treatment reduces oxidative stress and modifies inflammatory pathways to aid in the reduction of inflammation and the advancement of healing.

- **Increased Production of Collagen and Elastin:** Fibroblast activity is stimulated, which results in a rise in the production of these two important proteins for the health and elasticity of the skin.

- **Neuroprotection and Enhancement of Cognitive performance:** Red light treatment may promote brain health through strengthening cerebral blood flow, decreasing neuroinflammation, and improving cognitive performance, according to emerging studies.

Chapter Three

Technique on How to Begin Red Light Therapy Treatment

1. Selecting the Appropriate Equipment

• Device Types: Masks, lamps, panels, and handheld gadgets.

• Wavelengths, irradiance, coverage area, and safety certifications are important factors to take into account.

• Suggested Brands and Models: A summary of well-liked and dependable red light therapy equipment.

2. Setting Your Therapy Area

• Location: Choosing a

welcoming, easily accessible, and quiet space.

• Setting up: Making sure the area is tidy and distraction-free.

• Device positioning: arranging the device correctly for maximum exposure and impact.

3. Safety Procedures and Directives

• Eye Protection: It's critical to use goggles to shield eyes from bright light.

• Skin Sensitivity: Monitoring for negative responses and modifying exposure as necessary.

• Usage Instructions: Adhere to the advice and guidelines provided by the manufacturer for safe usage.

Method of Application

4. Direct and indirect and Applications

- **Direct Application:** For focused treatment, place the light source close to the skin.
- **Indirect Application:** To achieve wider exposure, use reflective surfaces or position the light further away.

5. **Duration and Frequency of Sessions**

- **Length of Session:** Usually lasting between five and twenty minutes.
- **Frequency:** Depending on the ailment being treated, the recommended frequency can range from everyday to several

times each week.

- **Consistency:** For best outcomes, it's critical to stick to a regular routine.

6. Using Red Light Therapy in conjunction with Other Therapies

- **Complementary Therapies:** Combining massage, physical therapy, and other treatments with red light therapy.
- **Skincare regimens:** For better skin benefits, combine topical treatments with red light therapy.
- **Physical fitness:** Combined with workout regimens for enhanced muscular performance and recuperation.

Advanced Technique

7. Specialized Interventions for Particular Illnesses

- **Skin Conditions:** psoriasis, wound healing, eczema, and acne.
- **Inflammation and Pain:** tendinitis, arthritis, and stiffness in the muscles.
- **Neurological Benefits:** Better mood and increased cognitive function.

8. Customize Protocol for individual needs

- **personalized Treatment Plans:** Evaluate each patient's needs and make necessary protocol adjustments.
- **Progress monitoring:** keeping

tabs on outcomes and modifying treatment as needed.

- **Consulting Professionals:** Asking medical professionals for guidance on complicated illnesses.

9. Including Red Light Therapy in Workplace Settings

- **Medical and Therapeutic Settings:** Utilize in physical therapy facilities, hospitals, and clinics.
- **Applications in Cosmetics and Aesthetics:** Including in wellness and beauty regimens.
- **Athletic training:** Used by trainers and sports teams to improve performance and recuperation.

Chapter Four

Application Techniques Comparing Indirect and Direct Applications

1. **Direct Application**

- **Proximity:** Keeping the light source a short distance—usually a few inches—from the skin.

- **Targeted Areas:** Concentrating on particular bodily parts, including the face, joints, or muscles, that require medical attention.

- **Intensity and Duration:** To ascertain the ideal intensity and duration for direct exposure, adhere to the device's specifications.

- **Techniques**
- **stationary treatment:** Maintaining a stationary light over the intended region is known as
- Moving Treatment: To cover a broader area, move the light slowly over the skin.

2. Indirect Application

- **Distance:** Place the light source a greater distance from the body—usually a few feet.
- **Broader Coverage:** offering a more comprehensive exposure to a greater number of body regions.
- **Diffuse Lighting:** To uniformly distribute light, employ reflective surfaces or angles.

- **Techniques**

Room Illumination: Passive exposure is enabled by using larger panels to illuminate a room or area.

Reflective Surfaces: To improve light distribution, place reflective materials all around the treatment area.

Duration and Frequency of Sessions

3. Duration of Session

- **Quick Sessions:** 5–10 minutes; good for first treatments or skin that is sensitive.

- **Standard Sessions:** 10–20 minutes are usually advised for the majority of applications.

- **Extended Sessions:** 20–30

minutes; ideal for persistent problems or deeper tissue penetration.

4. Frequency

- **Daily Usage:** For severe ailments or rigorous therapy regimens.
- **Several Times a Week:** Usually for upkeep and general wellness.
- **Weekly Use:** For long-term health advantages and preventive care.

5. Consistency

- **Regular Schedule:** For long-term advantages, it's critical to keep a regular schedule.
- **Tracking Progress:** Maintaining a record or log of

meetings and outcomes in order to keep an eye on advancements and modify procedures as necessary.

Chapter Five

Red Light Therapy in Combination with Other Therapies Treatment

6. Complementary Therapies

• **Physical therapy:** When coupled with manual therapies and physical exercises, it improves recovery and lessens discomfort.

• **Massage Therapy:** Applied either prior to or following massage treatments, it enhances relaxation and relieves muscle tension.

• **Chiropractic Care:** Using adjustments from the chiropractor to support spinal health and treat pain.

7. Skincare Schedules

- **Topical Treatments:** To enhance the effects of red light treatment for skincare, apply serums, creams, or lotions before or after.
- **facial Masks:** To improve skin tone and texture, use red light therapy masks intended for face treatments.
- **Anti-Aging Protocols:** For maximum benefits, combine with other anti-aging procedures including chemical peels or microdermabrasion.

8. physical Fitness

- **Pre-Workout:** To warm up muscles and lower the chance of injury, use red light treatment prior to activity.

- **post workout** Red light treatment can be applied post-workout to hasten recuperation and lessen discomfort in the muscles.
- **Performance Enhancement:** Increasing strength and endurance through training regimens that include red light treatment.

Advanced Methods
Targeted Treatment for Specific Condition

1. Skin Conditions
- **Acne:** Red light treatment reduces inflammation and

eliminates bacteria that cause acne. Treatment protocols often involve daily or every other-day sessions for a few weeks.

- **Psoriasis and eczema:** Regular, brief sessions can help reduce inflammation, redness, and itching.
- **Wound Healing:** Applying concentrated light therapy can hasten the healing of burns, cuts, and surgical wounds.

2. Inflammation and Pain

- **Arthritis:** Using near-infrared light to target the problematic areas, joint pain and stiffness can be reduced.
- **Tendonitis:** Direct use of red light promotes healing and

lessens discomfort in tendons.

- **Muscle Soreness:** Using red light therapy after exercise helps relieve delayed onset muscle soreness (DOMS).

3. Neurologists Benefits

- **Cognitive Enhancement:** Applying near-infrared light to the head to improve mental acuity and brain function.
- **Mood Improvement:** Regular exposure to red light can help reduce the symptoms of anxiety and despair.
- **Neurodegenerative Conditions:** By improving mitochondrial function in neural tissues, this supports treatment strategies for diseases like

Parkinson's and Alzheimer's.

Customizing Protocols for Individual Needs

4. **Personalized Treatment Plans**

- **Assessment:** Creating customized red light therapy regimens by assessing each person's health problems and aspirations.
- **Adjustment:** Changing frequency, length, and intensity in accordance with each person's response and development.
- **Holistic Approach:** Adding lifestyle elements to red light therapy, such as exercise, diet, and stress reduction.

5. Tracking Development

- **Monitoring Outcomes**: Preserving an exhaustive record of every session, encompassing the day, length, and observable impacts.
- **Modifying Protocols:** Changing treatment parameters in response to feedback and continuing outcomes.
- **Frequent Check-ins:** To guarantee the best results, schedule regular reviews with a therapist or healthcare professional.

6. Consulting with Specialists

- **Medical Guidance**: Consulting physicians or other experts for guidance regarding complicated or long-term ailments.

- **Therapeutic Support:** Including red light therapy into more comprehensive treatment regimens by collaborating with dermatologists, physical therapists, and chiropractors.
- **Professional Training:** Taking classes or workshops to expand on your understanding of red light therapy use.

Red Light Therapy's Integration Into Professional Practice

7. Health and Rehabilitation Environments

- **Clinics and hospitals:** Red light therapy is being used for wound healing, pain relief, and rehabilitation.

- **Physical Therapy Centers:** Improving the results of musculoskeletal disorders with the use of red light therapy.
- **Rehabilitation Programs:** Including red light therapy in surgical and injury rehabilitation regimens.

8. Applications in Cosmetics and Aesthetics

beauty salons and spas: Red light treatment is a service provided by beauty salons and spas to promote skin renewal and anti-aging.

Dermatology practices: Red light treatment is used to treat a variety of skin diseases and enhance the health of the skin.

Anti-aging clinics: Red light treatment can be used into full anti-aging regimens offered by anti-aging clinics.

9. Sports Instruction

sport team: Red light therapy is being used by sports teams to improve performance, reduce injuries, and hasten recovery.

- **Personal Trainers:** Including red light treatment in clients' training plans.
- **Recovery Centers:** Providing athletes and other active people with red light treatment as part of their recovery services.

Chapter Six

Benefits of red light therapy Skin Care and Beauty

1. Reducing Wrinkles and fine lines

• Red light therapy increases the creation of collagen and elastin by stimulating fibroblasts, which improves skin suppleness and minimizes the appearance of wrinkles.

• Better Texture: Promotes cell turnover and regeneration to improve the texture of the skin, resulting in firmer, smoother skin.

2. Treating Acne and other

skin condition

- **Anti-Inflammatory Effects:** Lowers inflammation brought on by psoriasis, eczema, and acne.
- **Antibacterial Properties:** Eliminates microorganisms that cause acne, assisting in the healing of outbreaks and averting more.
- **Healing and Scarring:** Promotes quicker healing of skin lesions and lessens the visibility of hyper pigmentation and scars.

3. Promoting Wound Healing and Scar Reduction

- **Enhanced Healing:** Encourages tissue repair and lowers inflammation to hasten the healing of wounds.

- **Remodeling Scar Tissue:** This process stimulates the growth of new, healthy tissue while destroying existing scar tissue to improve the look of scars.

Reduction of Pain and Inflammation

4. Techniques for Relieving Pain

- **Enhanced Blood Flow:** Encourages vasodilation, which improves blood flow to afflicted areas and lessens discomfort.
- **Endorphin Release:** Induces the body's natural pain-relieving hormone, endorphin release.

5. Circumstances Where Red Light Therapy Is Beneficial

- **Chronic Pain:** Reduces discomfort brought on by ailments such as fibromyalgia, arthritis, and persistent back pain.
- **Acute Injuries:** Quickens the healing process and lessens discomfort from sprains, strains, and fractures.

6. Testimonials and Case Studies

- **Patient Success Stories:** Actual accounts of people who used red light therapy to significantly reduce their pain and enhance their quality of life.
- **Clinical Trials:** A summary of studies showing red light therapy's effectiveness in treating

pain.

Muscle Recuperation and Optimal Performance

7. Advantages for Participants and Active People

- **Accelerated Recovery:** Lessens inflammation and discomfort in the muscles, enabling a speedier recovery period in between sessions.
- **Injury Prevention:** By preserving the health of muscles and joints, it helps to prevent injuries.

8. Applications for Before and After Exercise

- Pre-Workout: To warm up

muscles and enhance performance, use red light therapy prior to exercise.

- **Red light treatment** can be applied post-workout to minimize muscle soreness and hasten recovery.

9. Improving the Growth and Repair of Muscles

- **Enhanced Protein Synthesis**: Promotes the synthesis of proteins necessary for muscle growth and repair.
- **Lessened Muscle Damage:** Reduces the amount of oxidative stress and damage that intensive exercise causes to the muscles.

Cognitive Function and Mental Health

10. Impact on Stress and Mood

- **Mood Improvement:** By encouraging the release of serotonin and endorphins, this technique reduces the symptoms of anxiety and despair.

- **Stress Reduction:** Lower cortisol levels aid in stress management and enhance general health.

11. Potential Advantages for Mental Health Issues

- **Neuroprotection:** Maintains the health of the brain by shielding neurons from harm.

- **Cognitive Enhancement:** May

help with diseases like Parkinson's and Alzheimer's by enhancing memory, concentration, and cognitive function.

12. Research and Study Results

- **Clinical Evidence:** A summary of research showing red light therapy's beneficial effects on mental health and cognitive performance.

Anecdotal reports are first-hand narratives from people who have used red light therapy to improve their mental health.

Red light therapy has many advantages, including bettering

the health and appearance of the skin, relieving pain and inflammation, improving muscle recovery and performance, and being beneficial for athletes and physically active people. It also has favorable effects on mental health and cognitive function, with potential benefits for mood enhancement and neuroprotection. By being aware of these advantages and taking advantage of them, people can maximize their health and well-being through red light therapy.

Uses
Red Light Treatment in Medical Settings

1. Employed in clinics and hospitals

• Pain Management: For individuals with persistent pain issues, red light therapy can be incorporated into pain management programs.

• **Wound Care:** Pressure sores and diabetic ulcers can both be treated with red light therapy, both acute and chronic.

• **Post-Surgical Recovery:** Targeted red light treatment improves healing and lowers pain and inflammation following surgery.

2. Incorporation into Rehabilitation and Physical Therapy

- **Musculoskeletal Conditions**: Red light treatment is used to treat tendinitis, arthritis, and muscle strains in order to lessen discomfort and enhance function.
- **Rehabilitation Programs:** By encouraging tissue repair and lowering inflammation, these programs aid in the recuperation process following operations and injuries.

3. Patient Outcomes and Success Stories

- **Clinical Case Studies:** These provide particular examples of how red light treatment has considerably enhanced patient outcomes in healthcare environments.

- **Patient Testimonials:** Telling the tales of those who have recovered and found relief via red light therapy.

Chapter Seven

Red Light Therapy at Home

4. Practical tips for Home use

- **Setting Up:** Organizing your home so that red light treatment works well and safely, taking into account gadget location and available space.
- **Routine Development:** To guarantee continuous effects, red light treatment sessions should be established on a regular basis.

5. Common Personal

Electronics

- **Handheld Devices:** Small and lightweight choices for focused medical interventions.

Larger equipment such as panels and bulbs allow for greater coverage and longer, more intense sessions.

- **Masks and Wearables:** specialized gadgets made for targeted use and cosmetic treatments.

6. Diy solution and affordable option

- **Budget-Friendly Devices:** Locating reasonably priced, high-performing red light therapy equipment.

- **DIY Setups:** How to make

inexpensive lights and common materials into DIY red light treatment setups.

Pets Red Light Therapy

7. Advantages for Animal Well-being

- **Pain Relief:** Relieving pain and suffering in animals with injuries, arthritis, and other ailments.
- **Skin and Coat Health**: Treating conditions like dermatitis and hair loss to promote the health of a pet's skin and coat.

8. Typical Uses in Veterinary Medicine

- **Post-Surgical Recovery:** Improving recuperation and

minimizing discomfort following surgical operations.

- **Chronic problems:** Regular red light therapy sessions can help manage chronic problems in pets, such as hip dysplasia and arthritis.

9. Success Stories and Case Studies

- **Veterinary Case Studies:** Illustrative accounts of successful red light treatment implementations by veterinarians.
- **Pet Owner Testimonials:** Narratives from pet owners who have witnessed notable enhancements in the health and welfare of their animals.

Innovative and Future Applications

10. New Research and Its Possible Applications

- **Advanced Healing Applications:** Examining how red light therapy might be used to treat more complicated illnesses including diabetes and heart disease.
- **Treatments for Mental Health:** Investigating the application of red light therapy to ailments such as anxiety, depression, and cognitive decline.

11. Technological Progress

- **Device Innovations:** Red light treatment devices have

undergone advancements in terms of power, efficiency, and user-friendly features.

- **Smart Devices:** Red light therapy sessions can be tracked and customized with the use of smart technologies.

12. Red light therapy's prospects in the medical field

- **Personalized Medicine:** How red light treatment might be incorporated into healthcare regimens that are tailored to each patient's requirements and circumstances.

- **Wider Acceptance and Integration:** Red light therapy is becoming more widely acknowledged and incorporated into conventional medical and wellness procedures.

Note: Red light therapy has many uses in the medical field, at-home use, veterinary care, and future innovative treatments. In the medical field, it helps with pain management, wound care, and rehabilitation. For individuals, it provides useful and reasonably priced ways to incorporate red light therapy into everyday activities. Veterinary applications show substantial advantages for animal health, and new research and technological developments indicate exciting future prospects. By comprehending and utilizing these uses, people can maximize the advantages of red light therapy for a variety of health and wellness requirements.

Chapter Eight

Commonly Asked Questions
Generally Questions

First of all, what is red light therapy (RLT)?

• Response: Red light therapy (RLT) is a procedure that penetrates the skin using certain red and near-infrared light wavelengths to encourage a range of cellular rejuvenation and healing benefits.

2. How is red light therapy applied?

• Response: Red light therapy (RLT) boosts the synthesis of ATP, the energy currency of cells, by stimulating the skin's mitochondria through low-level exposure to red or near-infrared light. This process improves cellular function and encourages healing and regeneration.

3. How safe is red light therapy?

• In general, red light treatment is safe when used appropriately; it is non-invasive and does not use UV radiation, which can cause skin damage. Nevertheless, it is crucial to adhere to manufacturer instructions and get individualized guidance from a healthcare professional.

Technical Question

4. Which wavelengths work best for red light therapy?

- The range of 600–700 nanometers (nm) for red light and 700–1100 nm for near-infrared light is the most effective for red light treatment. These wavelengths are well absorbed by the skin and tissues, encouraging therapeutic effects.

5. How much time should pass between Red Light Therapy sessions?

- Response: Depending on the ailment being treated and the

treatment region, sessions can last anywhere from five to twenty minutes. It is crucial to adhere to the manufacturer's recommendations for the device in order to achieve the best possible outcomes.

6. How frequently must I to apply red light therapy?

• The number of red light therapy sessions can vary, but consistency is essential to getting the best outcomes. Many protocols suggest using red light therapy everyday or every other day for the first period, followed by maintenance sessions several times a week.

Uses and Application

7. Is it possible to utilize red light therapy at home?

• The answer is that there are a lot of devices that may be used at home, such as masks, panels, and handheld devices. To ensure safe and efficient treatment, it's crucial to select a high-quality gadget and carefully follow the instructions.

8. Is it possible to use Red Light Therapy to any body part?

• The majority of the body, including the face, neck, back, joints, and muscles, can benefit from red light therapy. However, delicate areas like the eyes should be shielded during treatment.

9. Do safety glasses have to be worn when receiving red light therapy?

• To protect your eyes from excessive light exposure, using protective eyewear is advised. This is especially true when utilizing powerful devices or treating areas close to the eyes.

Advantages and Efficiency

10. What ailments is Red Light Therapy effective in treating?

• Response: Red light treatment is beneficial for a number of ailments, such as pain and inflammation (arthritis, muscular soreness), skin problems (acne, wrinkles, scars), and general health (better mood, sharper cognitive function).

11. How long does red light therapy take to show results?

• Response: Depending on the ailment being treated and the patient, results can vary. While some people show dramatic improvements after just a few sessions, others may need to utilize the treatment consistently for several weeks.

12. Is it possible to combine Red Light Therapy with other forms of treatment?

• In order to improve overall outcomes, red light therapy can be used in conjunction with other therapies such topical skincare products, physical therapy, and wellness regimens.

Advanced Question

13. Is there a period of recovery following Red Light Therapy sessions?

• Response: Red light therapy sessions usually don't require any recovery period; you can get back to your regular activities right away.

14. Does red light therapy have any negative side effects?

• Response: While moderate skin redness or irritation are unusual side effects, they can occur and normally go away quickly. It's best to start with shorter sessions so you can monitor your skin's response and make any adjustments.

15. Can mental health problems be helped by Red Light Therapy?

• Response: Red light therapy may benefit mental health; it can lessen symptoms of anxiety and depression and improve cognitive function, according to emerging research. Nevertheless, it should be used in addition to professional mental health care, not as a substitute for it.

www.ingramcontent.com/pod-product-compliance
Lightning Source LLC
Chambersburg PA
CBHW071958210526
45479CB00003B/988